INDIGESTION:
ITS CAUSE AND CURE

INDIGESTION:
ITS CAUSE AND CURE

JOHN HENRY CLARKE M.D.,

AMERICAN EDITION

Revised and Enlarged by the Author

From the Fifth English Edition

GYAN

Published by

GYAN

Gyan Publishing House
5, Ansari Road
Daryaganj, New Delhi-110002
Phone: 011-47034999, 9811692060
E-mail: books@gyanbooks.com

Distribution Network
gyanbooks.com
India, USA, Canada, UK, Australia, France

ISBN : 978-81-212-6548-5 (PB)
First Published, 1900

2nd Impression 2022

Printed at: Gyan Press, Delhi.

INDIGESTION: ITS CAUSE AND CURE
Author: JOHN HENRY CLARKE

INDIGESTION:
ITS CAUSES AND CURE.

BY

JOHN H. CLARKE, M. D.,

FELLOW OF THE BRITISH HOMŒOPATHIC SOCIETY; EXTRA-ORDINARY MEMBER OF THE ROYAL MEDICAL SOCIETY OF EDINBURGH; CONSULTING PHYSICIAN TO THE LONDON HOMŒOPATHIC HOSPITAL; AUTHOR OF "THE PRESCRIBER," ETC.

AMERICAN EDITION.

Revised and Enlarged by the Author,

From the Fifth English Edition.

1900

CONTENTS.

PREFACE TO THE FIFTH ENGLISH EDITION.

The continued popularity of this treatise, as evidenced by the exhaustion of another edition, is a gratifying circumstance in itself, and at the same time it enables me to keep it thoroughly up to date. In the present revised edition will be found much additional matter, including several new cases, which I hope will still further increase the usefulness of the work.

JOHN H. CLARKE.

PREFACE TO AMERICAN EDITION.

In presenting this little work to American Homœopathic readers, I can only express a hope that it may find as gratifying a reception on the western side of the Atlantic as it has done on this. Five editions have already been called for, and as the last was issued little more than a year ago I have not found it necessary to make any extensive alterations. At the same time I have gone carefully over the work and have been able to incorporate a considerable amount of new matter.

JOHN H. CLARKE.

30 Clarges Street, Piccadilly,
London, W.

June, 1899.

FROM THE PREFACE TO THE FIRST EDITION.

Considering the enormous influence the human stomach has exercised on the history of the world and of individuals, it is astonishing that people are so little careful how they treat it, and what they put into it. But for the stomach, as every one knows, there would be little of the world's work done. "If any man will not work, neither shall he eat," is the apostle's rendering of the primal curse, "In the sweat of thy face shalt thou eat bread." And certain it is that but for the stomach and its demands there would be a very great scarcity of workers. Nor does the doing of the work alone depend on the stomach's wants;, the quality of it also depends very much on the stomach's condition. When a man cannot eat a mouthful of food without suffering acute misery, it is impossible for him to work with the pleasure that the best work demands, or to take a just and charitable view of his fellow-creatures; and when the man happens to be one of the rulers or leaders of men, the consequences may be far-reaching.

It becomes, therefore, a matter of the first importance in life to give the stomach fair play. In the following pages, after describing the normal process of digestion, I go on to sketch the various deviations from the normal to which the process is liable, and to show how they may be avoided, and how cured.

I have illustrated the treatment of the various kinds of indigestion by narrating the treatment of actual cases. It will be seen that the treatment is of several kinds.

In some cases of acute indigestion, the best remedy is to abstain from food for twenty-four hours, and take no medicine at all. In most cases the regulation of the diet, and the time at which it should be taken, is a matter of the first importance. But there are many cases in which this is not enough; and in almost all cases it may be usefully supplemented. It often happens that the conditions of life are such that the active causes of indigestion are operating all the time, and no change in regimen is possible. What is to be done in these cases? A melancholy-wise shake of the head on the part of the physician does not provide much help, and though this is often all the sufferer receives, it is because the physician does not know his business.

There is much to be done; but he who knows not Hahnemann and Homœopathy will fail to do it.

It is just here that Homœopathy shines with such conspicuous lustre beside Old Physic. By means of its powerful and yet innocuous medicines it can work out cures when Allopathy must stand helplessly by, or make matters worse by giving drugs that are almost certain to do harm.

After narrating my cases, I shall devote a chapter to the diet treatment of indigestion, and then, in a final chapter, I shall give a list of the medicines which are most useful in the disease, with the particular indications for their use.

CHAPTER I.

DIGESTION.

THE process of digestion commences immediately that food is taken into the mouth. Before food can be converted into blood, it is necessary that it be reduced to a liquid or semi-liquid state. All solid foods, therefore, must be broken down in the first instance to fine particles, and for this purpose the teeth are provided. Solids may be swallowed unmasticated, it is true, and the strong digestive juices are capable of digesting them, but this power is made much more certain and easy if the food has been first finely ground by the teeth. But the teeth have another function. In the cheeks and under the tongue are the salivary glands, the ducts of which convey the saliva into the mouth, and one function of the teeth is to mix the food thoroughly with saliva at the same time that they grind it small. The leading action of the saliva is on the starchy elements of the food, which are converted by it from insoluble starch into soluble grape-sugar. In this way solid food is prepared for its passage into the stomach, which is the organ of digestion *par excellence.*

The stomach may be defined as an organ for the reception, at proper intervals, of food and water. I say "water," rather than "drink," because whatever drink is taken, it is the water which is the essential thirst-quenching part of it. The stomach, when it has received the food, does not complete the digestion of it, as many people imagine, but it does by far the largest share of the work in liquefying the food and reducing it to a condition in which it can be absorbed. It is lined with a mucous membrane richly supplied with glands of a special kind, which secrete a very powerful acid fluid. This fluid acts chemically on the food taken, breaking it up and reducing it to a pulp. It also contains the substance "pepsin," which acts in a peculiar way like a ferment, converting all the albuminous foods, such as meats of all kinds, into "peptones" which can be absorbed, in the same way that saliva converts starch into grape-sugar. Besides the mucous coat there is a muscular coat, with fibres running in two directions,—from end to end, lengthways of the organ, and circularly, all round it. By these two sets of fibres the food is moved about when the stomach is full, until it has all come in contact with the mucous membrane and been submitted to the action of the gastric juice. When thoroughly mixed with this, the whole being reduced to a grey, semi-fluid mass, it is ready to be passed on into the bowels. There it meets with the bile, the pancreatic juice, and the secretions of the intestinal glands and mucous membrane; and as each different secretion acts on it, some portion of it is rendered ready to be taken up by the absorbent vessels called lacteals which abound in the intestines. In the lacteals it is a fluid and looks like milk. After passing through the abdominal glands, where it undergoes some further preparation, the fluid is at last collected from all the lacteals into one large duct (the *thoracic duct*) and poured into the current of the blood.

This is the *primary* digestion, and that alone with which I concern myself in the present treatise;

but there is also a *secondary* digestion, to which I will briefly refer. All the tissues of the body are in a state of ebb and flow. Where life is there is no standing still; everything is in a state of motion and change. The tissues once built up from the food no sooner reach their perfection and perform their function than they begin to decay and make room for more. Some tissues change more rapidly than others—the soft tissues more rapidly than the hard, but all change and break down into their elements. The *secondary* digestion consists in the absorption of these decomposed elements by the lymphatic vessels and glands, the elimination of those elements which are entirely waste, and the recomposition of those that are still utilizable into blood and new tissues.

This process is one of vast importance, and one which is easily deranged. Some people naturally have a more active secondary digestion than others, and these are generally thin. Tissue-change goes on rapidly, and it matters little how much they eat, they can never fatten. In spite of their spareness they have generally great vital heat, and are of an active, nervous, and restless temperament. Others, on the contrary, eat little, but grow constantly fat. With them the process is slow; the tissues burn away (for it is essentially a burning process) less rapidly, and they are of a quieter, more easy-going disposition—lymphatic or phlegmatic. But when there is not merely slow tissue-change, but, in addition to this, a defect in the carrying off of the effete matters from the tissues, then we have various kinds of diseases arising as the effete matters accumulate in the system. If it is lactic acid, we have rheumatism; if the predominating substance is uric acid, we have gout. These are, in general, diseases of the *secondary* digestion. It is of course possible, and, indeed, most common, to have defects of the two digestions combined, but they are distinct things nevertheless.

I have said that the secondary digestion is easily interfered with.

All lowering influences put a check on it. Too great exposure to cold, for instance, will stop it, as in the chill which sets up rheumatic fever. Alcohol, tea, coffee, opium, tobacco, check it; hence some of the diseases that spring from over-indulgence in these as articles of ordinary consumption. Of course, it will be easily understood that the two digestions act and react on each other; and it must not be forgotten that the above-mentioned substances powerfully affect the primary digestion, and may disorder that as well as the secondary.

Having explained this much, I will return to a consideration of the stomach, for that is the organ which is chiefly concerned with what is popularly understood by "indigestion," and is, in fact, the most important of the digestive organs. If the stomach is in good condition the chances are that the rest of the organs of digestion are in good condition also, and if these are not sound, the stomach is pretty sure to feel it, and let its owner know.

CHAPTER II.

CAUSES OF INDIGESTION.

BEFORE proceeding further I wish to be clear about terms. Medical terms are often confusing to non-medical readers, who attach differences of meaning to different terms when they are simply two names for the same thing. A familiar instance of this is the case of the terms "scarlatina" and "scarlet fever." The first is supposed to represent a mild form of the second. But they are used absolutely indifferently by medical men, the most malignant cases being called scarlatina, just as the mildest cases are called scarlet fever, and *vice versa*. There is the same distinction made by some people between "indigestion" and "dyspepsia." It is a distinction without a difference; both are names (indigestion, Latin; and dyspepsia, Greek) for identically the same condition, and I use them indifferently. I am sorry if I must rob some poor sufferer of the little consolation he has been able to obtain from the supposition that his complaint is not vulgar "indigestion," but a more refined something named "dyspepsia," but it must be done, for they are merely different names for the same thing.

A great deal might be profitably

written on the art of eating. Hurrying over meals, paradoxical as it may sound to say so, is the most extravagant waste of time. The teeth cannot do their proper share of mastication unless they have sufficient time to do it in ; the food is passed into the stomach in an unprepared state, and the lack of mental quiet prevents the stomach from expending a proper amount of energy on its duties. A meal-time should be a time of mental and bodily rest to all but the digestive faculties. Another point in the art of eating is the avoidance of drinking much during a meal. The practice of washing down every mouthful with a drink, whether of water, wine, lemonade, or what not, is exceedingly bad. It dilutes and weakens the action of the digestive juices, and almost certainly leads to dyspepsia. A good drink, if thirsty, shortly before a meal, or a little time after it, is the best arrangement; though a draught in the pauses between the courses need not be objected to. But food should never be "washed down."

A healthy stomach is able to digest anything in an ordinary way that is called food. Its power is not strictly limited to the digesting of "wholesome" food, but it has a margin of over-power, which allows it to undertake luxuries like mince pies, roast pork, and confectionery. The happy possessor of such an organ should enjoy what he eats and be thankful, and think little or nothing about his stomach. Only he must not transgress his margin. For the strongest stomach may be ruined if it is tried beyond its powers, and if its possessor uses it as a receptacle for things that please his palate, rather than for those which sustain his body. But if he makes the latter his main object, and only indulges his palate now and then, his stomach will take it all very good-naturedly, and no harm will be done.

The three grand requirements of every stomach are—proper food, proper quantity of food, and proper rest.

It does not matter how wholesome the food may be if there is not enough of it, or if there is too much, the stomach will resent it. Or, if the quantity as well as the quality be right, and if it be given irregularly, at improper intervals, allowing no time for the stomach to recover itself after its last digestive effort, indigestion will result.

A large number of the cases of indigestion we meet with arise from violation of these three cardinal rules. But not all. The stomach may be disordered when there is no complaint to be made whatever as to the treatment of the stomach itself. For instance, in all fevers and acute inflammations the digestion is more or less interfered with, though the stomach may not be originally at fault. Whatever damages the vitality of the blood, either in the way of blood-poisoning, or by its becoming watery and thin, impairs the power of digestion. Working in ill-ventilated offices with gas, or at poisonous trades, as in the case of cardboard boxmakers, paper-hangers and stainers, and artificial florists, who inhale arsenic, and plumbers who work with lead,—any of these conditions may set up indigestion. Improper habits of body, as neglect of open-air exercise, and excesses of every kind, will bring on a very inveterate form of indigestion. Inherited delicacy of any kind, whether consumptive, rheumatic, or gouty, will sometimes manifest itself in indigestion apart from any want of care on the patient's part. Finally, mental causes must not be omitted from the list. "Laugh and grow fat" is a very old adage and a very true one. When the mind is ill at ease the stomach cannot work as it ought, and the face grows haggard and lean and the muscles lax. Worry is one great cause of indigestion.

CHAPTER III.

FOOD AND DRINK.

WHAT is a food? This is not quite so easy a question to answer as some people might suppose. Any substance which is capable of being digested and converted into the tissues of the body is a food. This is the scientific definition; but there are many substances which have been eaten, and which have actually helped to sustain life under emergencies, which we are not in the habit of looking upon as food in an ordinary way. For instance, in times of siege, leather has been actually eaten by starving people, but we don't consider leather a food. Therefore in practical life it is only those substances which contain a considerable amount of digestible material that are to be regarded as foods.

Moreover, the question, What is a food? can only be answered by each individual for himself. What is a food to one man is not necessarily a food to another. Such an innocent thing as mutton, for instance, would be said by most people to be good food for everybody, and yet I know those to whom the least bit of mutton is dangerous poison. Many people can eat mackerel and enjoy it without feeling any after-effect; in others the smallest portion of it will set up choleraic symptoms. Some people are so sensitive that fish of any kind will cause violent nettlerash. I have known others who are sure to have a severe fit of asthma if they even smell roast hare. Finally, some people are poisoned if they eat rice, and can detect its presence in beer by their symptoms when merely a few grains of it have been put into the beer at the time of bottling.

In our definition of "food," therefore, we must make room for exceptions; it is not all substances containing nutriment that are food for everybody.

Foods are divided into two kinds, —those in which the nitrogenous or albuminous elements predominate, and those which contain the carbon elements in the greater proportion.

To the nitrogen class belong lean of meat, cheese, French beans, peas, lentils; whereas the carbon class is represented by fat of meat, butter, farinaceous foods, sugar, potatoes, and bread. The only perfect food is milk, containing both elements in good proportions. Eggs also contain both elements, but they are not such a perfect food as milk, as they do not contain the necessary salts in solution as milk does. Of course there are other things in foods besides these two predominating elements, though these serve to usefully classify them. And it must not be supposed that the members of one class have none of the elements characteristic of the other. It is only the proportion which serves to distinguish them ; meat contains carbon as well as nitrogen, and bread contains nitrogen as well as carbon. Nor are the members of the same class alike, rice and bread are both in the carbon class, but rice contains less nitrogen than bread.

There is another food element the importance of which has been rightly emphasized by Dr. Lahmann, namely, food-salts. These are contained in milk in the right proportion as regards other food elements, and also in the right relative proportions among themselves. Soda, potash, and lime salts are the principal. These are contained in the various fruits and vegetables in sufficient excess to make up for the deficiency of them in meats, and pulse foods, such as peas, beans, and lentils. It is important that vegetables should be cooked by steaming, as the common practice of boiling them boils most of their salts out of them and common table-salt does not make up for the deficiency.

Cow's milk contains .7 per cent. of food-salts, which have the following percentage composition:

Potash, K_2O.	Soda, Na_2O.	Lime, Ca O.	Magnesia, Mg. O.	Oxide of Iron, Fe_2O_3.	Phosphoric Acid, P_2O_5.	Sulphuric Acid, S. O_3.	Silicic Acid, Si O_2.	Chlorine, C. S.
24.67	9.70	22.05	3.05	.53	28.45	.30	.04	14.28

Meat, white flour, potato, and pea contain very much less than the proper proportion of soda, lime, and chlorine than the standard of milk. Spinach, cabbage-lettuce, and carrot contain more than the standard. Apple and strawberry contain more than the standard of soda but less of lime. This shows the necessity of plenty of fresh fruits and green vegetables in the dietary of a meat-eating people. The use of common table-salt is no substitute for the lack of the right food-salts. Chloride of sodium is more of a stimulant than a food. It renders too rapid the passage of fluid from the tissues and causes an abnormal thirst. Salted meats are not such valuable foods as fresh meats; and for this reason. Three-fourths of the weight of fresh meat consists of water; but in contact with salt fresh meat loses some of its water, which passes into the urine and carries with it a considerable part of the effective organic and inorganic constituents of the meat (Gorup-Besanez). A similar process of "pickling" goes on in the bodies of those who eat excessively of salt. Another effect of over-indulgence in salt is the creation of acidity.*

Food, then to be satisfactory, must contain all of these elements; and the proportions should be about

* "Natural Hygiene," H. Lahmann, M. D., London: Swan Sonnenschein.

fifteen of the carbon (fat and sugar), and five of the nitrogen class (albumen), and one of salts. It is in order to keep the proportion between carbon and nitrogen that potatoes are taken with meat, and are better for that purpose than bread, which itself contains much of the nitrogenous elements. Cheese by itself is much too strong a food, and needs to be taken with bread, and perhaps butter as well.

Proper food, then, which I have said is the first requisite for the healthy stomach, consists of food-substances combined in proper proportions according to their nature, and, of course,—if cooked at all—properly cooked.

There is much dispute about

alcohol, as to whether it is a food or not in the proper sense of the word. If it be a food it is an uncommonly poor one. It is a carbohydrate, that is certain, and it is capable of being absorbed into the blood; but it no sooner gets there than every organ does its best to get rid of it, and if any of it undergoes a change in the blood, it can only be a very small proportion. It is a safe rule to make, never to consider anything as a food when there is any doubt about whether it is a food or not. There are plenty of things about which there is no doubt. Let these be taken as food, and if the doubtful articles are taken at all, let it be for some other reason, and not with the idea of nourishing the body.

Alcohol brings me to the question of drinks. Actually there is only one drink—water. Beer, tea, coffee, and the rest, are drinks, it is true, but they owe their property of thirst-quenching to the water they contain, not to the substances which flavour them. Milk is a drink, but it contains so much food, which becomes solid as soon as it enters the stomach, that it should only be taken as a drink at meal-times by those who are not able to take much solid food. It is well, as mentioned in the previous chapter, not to drink much of any liquid during a meal, but to take a good draught before it, or after it is over.

Some people have a great distaste for cold water, and some cannot digest it. For them *hot* water or toast-water may be substituted, when other drinks are objectionable.

The second great requisite for the stomach that I pointed out, is —Proper quantity of food.

The stomach requires a certain mass of food for it to work on. A healthy stomach will have nothing to do with essences or condensed foods; it requires bulk in order that its muscular coat may have something to grasp and contract on, and its secretion something to mix with. It is for this reason that the starchy foods, like potatoes, are the best to eat with meat, because the latter contains nutriment in so condensed a form that substances less rich must be added to make up sufficient bulk. When foods are prescribed in small quantity, and in light form, it is because the stomach is in an abnormal condition.

This leads me to speak of the third requisite—Proper rest.

When the stomach has dealt with a meal, pouring out its secretion, and by means of its muscular action reducing it to a proper state for further digestion in the intestines, it passes it on. Then the stomach has rest, and the other organs take up the work. The effort it has gone through is no light one, and it needs time to recover itself. If this time of rest is broken by subsidiary meals, or indulgence in confectionery, the stomach resents it, and the result is indigestion. Unless under special circumstances, no food whatever should be taken between meals, and a good five hours should be allowed between one meal and another. Three meals a day—at 8, 1, and 7 o'clock—is the best arrangement in an ordinary way. The middle meal should be very light if much active brain-work has to be done in the afternoon. In the morning the stomach is most vigorous, and a substantial meal can be taken then, though active work must be begun soon after. In the evening the powers of the body are more exhausted by the day's exertions, and yet a substantial meal can be taken at that time, as it is followed by a period of rest and relaxation.

To those in delicate health rest of

body, before and after food is almost as essential as rest of stomach. The robust may sit down to a hearty repast immediately after fatiguing employment. Not so the delicate: for them rest is necessary both before a meal and after. I have known invalids unable to take the lightest meal without suffering indigestion, if they took it immediately after the seemingly slight fatigue of dressing; whereas, if they rose a little earlier, so as to give themselves a quarter of an hour's rest before the meal-time, they ate with more appetite and digested their food without trouble.

CHAPTER IV.

INDIGESTION AFTER ITS KINDS.

1. *From Indigestible Food.*

WHEN a small boy strays into an orchard before the fruit is quite ripe, and indulges his appetite without staying to reflect, he is apt to experience an attack of indigestion of the simplest kind. The food he has eaten is not digested, but remains in his stomach like an irritating foreign body. If he is discovered in time, the simplest process is to give him an emetic of salt-and-water or mustard-and-water, and so get rid of it in this way. But if it has already had time to pass into the bowels, other measures will be needed. The symptoms he experiences are sharp pains in the upper part of the body or about the navel, and even cramp and spasms which may go on to general convulsions. Stone fruit before it is ripe will cause the same symptoms.

Those who have reached mature years are generally more discriminating in their diet, but every little while they may forget themselves. Perhaps it is some favourite dish which they know does not agree with them, but which they cannot resist, and then they know what to expect. The symptoms vary according to the food that has caused the indigestion. Nuts cause pains in the stomach* and chest. Fat food, especially fat pork, causes nausea and vomiting, with moist white tongue. This is frequently accompanied by pains in the body and diarrhœa.

Food may be indigestible under some conditions, and digestible under others. If a person in a state of

*Throughout this treatise I use the word "Stomach" in the anatomical sense, meaning the organ which receives the food as soon as it is swallowed. The stomach lies in the upper part of the abdominal cavity, more on the left side than on the right, which is occupied by the liver. The stomach is protected by the lowest ribs on the left side, and many of the pains arising in the stomach are felt in the chest. In common speech the "Stomach" means the whole of the abdomen, but I do not use it in this sense.

exhaustion sits down to a hearty meal, even though the food is nothing but what he is used to, he will not be able to digest it. In all such states the very lightest food should be taken until the bodily powers are restored, which usually happens after a sleep. Some people can eat hot meat very well, but not cold meat, and to them cold meat is an indigestible food. The explanation of this is that in cold meat the albuminous and gelatinous parts are set, whereas in hot meat they are fluid, and these are more easily acted on by the digestive juices; moreover, cold meat must become warm in the stomach before it can be digested, and this absorbs a certain amount of the stomach's vital energy. Pains in the chest and intestines, flatulence, and great distress, are the penalty of want of due care on these points.

Under the same heading of indigestion from indigestible food must come those cases due to defective teeth. When the teeth are faulty and cannot masticate the food properly before it is swallowed, it reaches the stomach ill-prepared, and sets up indigestion which is apt to become chronic. The remedy in this case is to consult a dentist, and if he cannot put matters right, the food—that is, the solid part of it—will have to be passed through a sausage machine and so chewed artificially.

2. *From excessive Indulgence in good Food.*

It is just as possible to injure the digestion with good food as with bad, if too much of it is taken. By a process of training, the stomach can become developed out of proportion to the rest of the body, and then large quantities of food can be taken without any active symptoms of indigestion. The stomach becomes to the gourmand what the athlete's limbs are to him —capable of an amount of exertion beyond the powers of other men. But over-development is not good in any part of the body, be it muscle or be it stomach; and the gourmnad pays the penalty before long. His powerful digestion lays up more pabulum than he requires; he grows in bulk without growing in strength, and is one day seized with a fit of gout,—he is fortunate if it attacks his toe and not some vital organ, or the stomach itself. Gouty dyspepsia is one of the most troublesome kinds to treat. Gout may be inherited as well as acquired, so it is not always the sufferer's own fault. There is in cases of gouty dyspepsia much acidity, flatulence, pain, and constipation.

3. *From Alcohol.*

The man who drinks excessively of beer loses consciousness, and has an acute attack of indigestion and vomiting. The vomiting relieves his stomach, a few hours' sleep restoring his senses, and after a day's indisposition he is well. But one who habitually indulges in beer and not necessarily to such excess, will have chronic dyspepsia of a different kind. Alcohol acts on both the primary and the secondary digestion, and the action of beer is to relax all the tissues of the body. The beer-drinker gradually becomes of the "flabby" or "sodden" type, probably pale and rather fat, and his digestion also becomes flabby and slow, and the tongue is large and yellow-coated, and there is much flatulence. Those who live active lives in the open air in the country do not show the effects so soon as those who live in towns and get little exercise.

Wine and spirits act somewhat differently. They do not cause so much puffiness as beer, but they redden the skin more, causing dilatation of the small blood-vessels, especially of the nose. Often there is pallor of the rest of the face, leaving the nose only red. There is in general wasting of the tissues of the body.

One marked symptom of the alcoholic dyspepsia—and this applies to all kinds, whether from beer, wine, or spirits—is sickness in the morning. There is bad appetite at any time, but in the morning, before anything has been taken, there is vomiting, of mucus generally. The tongue is tremulous, and there is a tremor through the body; flatulence and constipation generally accompany this kind.

4. *From Tobacco.*

The first attempts to smoke are almost always attended with an acute attack of indigestion, deathly nausea, and vomiting. But habitual over-indulgence in tobacco causes dyspepsia of a different kind. In the most aggravated form it is characterized by perpetual sickness; no food can be retained, and at this time, smoking, and even the smell of tobacco, is intolerable. In the less severe cases it takes the form of acidity, heartburn, pain after taking food, sinking sensation at the pit of the stomach, and generally constipation.

5. *From Tea.*

It would be difficult to say which is the greater cause of indigestion —alcohol or tea. It is true people don't often get drunk with the cup that "not inebriates" (though there has been one case reported, in which a woman who *ate* tea suffered from delirium tremens in consequence), but they do often get dyspepsia. In the tea dyspepsia the nervous symptoms predominate. There is more pain at the stomach than sickness or vomiting, the tongue is not so large and flabby as with beer-drinkers, and the subjects of it suffer more from what is called "nerves." They are always on high tension, easily startled, sleep little, and have no appetite for anything but—tea. They want tea always; it is the only thing that relieves the "sinking" they complain of (itself a consequence of the tea). They suffer much from low spirits.

6. *From Cold.*

Few things stop digestion so soon as lowering the bodily temperature. A cold bath soon after a meal arrests the process completely, and is very apt to cause dangerous symptoms. A drive in cold air with insufficient wraps will cause symptoms of indigestion, chiefly pains in the stomach, and flatulence. The next meal gives great pain, and it takes some time for the stomach to recover from the injury.

7. *From Bad Air.*

When many hours of the twenty-four are passed in air that is spent, heated by gas, or polluted by the breath of human beings which cannot escape, it is impossible for the digestion to go on properly. The stomach, as well as the rest of the body, loses its proper vitality; the digestive fluids are not able to transform the food eaten; and, for want of proper oxygen in the blood, the secondary digestion is imperfectly performed. The results are wasting and pain.

8. *From Vinegar.*

Some persons who have a tendency to grow fat take to drinking vinegar, in order to prevent such a dreadfully unbecoming calamity falling upon them. Many have succeeded by this means in bringing about "vinegar-consumption," and dying of it. Others have gained their object at the price of no worse a disease than ruined digestion. Constant acidity, pain after food, flatulence, flushing of the face, great thinness, are the leading symptoms of vinegar dyspepsia.

9. *From Tight-lacing.*

Another vanity for which many women pay dearly is a wasp-waist. Wherein the beauty of this anatomical enormity consists it is difficult to discover, and it must be classed along with the foot deforming custom of the Chinese, and the head flattening of some tribes of North American Indians. The organs of digestion resent it, and show their resentment by painting the nose red, and torturing the offender whenever she attempts to put food into the stomach without leaving it proper room. Constipation is usually one result of this.

10. *From Nervous Debility.*

Some of the most inveterate cases of indigestion arise from weakness of the nervous system. This may be brought on in many ways. It may be due to nervous strain or worry of business. It may arise from fright, mental shock, or anxiety. Much more frequently it arises from evil habits and abuse of the organs of generation. One vicious boy at school will often corrupt numbers of others, and so the disease will spread like an infection, bearing fruit before long in the loss of all manly qualities, and in sufferings of a most distressing kind connected with the process of digestion. These cases, like most of the others, are curable, but they need much care, and, of course, a *sine quâ non* is the abandonment of the habits that have brought about the disorder.

11. *From Bloodlessness.*

Young girls between 12 and 20

are very frequently affected with a disease commonly called "green-sickness." This is chiefly a fault of digestion, primary or secondary, or both, but it is also a fruitful cause of digestive troubles. There is almost complete loss of appetite, constant nausea, frequent vomiting. Usually, also, there is great weakness and constipation. When the condition is attended by violent pains at the stomach after all food, it is not easy to distinguish between simple indigestion and ulceration of the stomach. This is usually declared by vomiting of blood in quantity, which never takes place in ordinary indigestion, and is rarely, if ever, absent at some period of ulceration.

12. *Medicinal.*

Many a sufferer from indigestion traces his troubles to the prescriptions of his doctor. It is one of the commonest experiences of medical life, to find digestion ruined by strong drugs given for other complaints. Others owe it not to their doctors, but to their own efforts to cure themselves with drugs. Probably, in the first instance, it has been a slight attack of indigestion from indiscretion in diet, for which the offender has purchased a drug according to his own fancy. Then the drug has set up symptoms of its own, for which he has taken more drugs. More symptoms have followed, and the drugging has become a habit which he has not been able to break off. Palliatives, like *Carbonate of Soda* and *Bismuth*, are responsible for many cases of confirmed dyspepsia, and *Iron*, *Mercury*, and acids for many more. The symptoms in these cases vary according to the drugs which have caused them.

13. *Constitutional.*

A depraved or disordered constitutional state is often answerable for chronic indigestion. Persons who inherit a tendency to skin disease frequently find that when their skin is affected their digestion is good, and *vice versa*. This is what Hahnemann called *psora*. In such cases, the only treatment that is of any permanent service is one which is directed to the constitution as a whole. The indigestion is only one symptom of many.

Indigestion is frequently a manifestation of the consumptive tendency which is one of the branches of *Psora*, and in such cases *Tuberculinum* or *Bacillinum* often greatly assists the cure. Occasional doses may be given inter-currently with the symptomatically indicated remedy.

The *hydrogenoid* constitution of Grauvogl is answerable for many indigestive troubles. The symptoms of this are an extraordinary sensitiveness to cold, damp, and barometrical changes. The persons are always chilly. Residence by water, in valleys, or forests, passing storms, and change of weather brings on attacks of illness, which takes various forms. Sometimes it is general malaise, with no definite symptoms, only the patient feels wretched, good for nothing. At other times it is an attack of asthma or ague. Certain kinds of food disagree with them, such as melons, cucumbers, mushrooms, bard-boiled eggs, watery fruits, fish, and sometimes milk. They are generally pale, and have cold feet. They are better in summer than in winter, and are relieved when they perspire. This constitution may be inherited or acquired. It often follows malarial poisoning. The particular form of indigestion attending this constitution is marked by pains in the stomach, water-brash eructations of odourless gas, often brought on by eating watery fruits or vegetables and vegetable acids. There is distaste for animal food, though the appetite is often good.

Vaccination often leaves behind it a depraved state of the constitution with many hydrogenoid symptoms, and the development of abdominal flatulence. *Thuja* meets most of these cases.

14. *From Gout.*

Chronic gout is answerable for much indigestion. It takes a great variety of forms and is often attended with pains in the joints or affections of the skin. There is loss of appetite, acidity, tendency to flatulence, generally constipation. Gouty persons are inclined to the formation of fat in spite of small appetite. This is in consequence of insufficient oxidation of the tissues. They have nearly always a great desire for the open air.

Some persons who are constitutionally dyspeptic always suffer from an attack when the wind is in the east.

In addition to the above-named, there are cases of dyspepsia arising from causes which cannot easily be classed, and some which seem to arise from no discoverable cause, and which are hence termed self-causing, or, in the medical phrase, "idiopathic."

In the following chapter I shall describe the treatment of the different kinds of indigestion, and shall relate a number of typical cases.

CHAPTER V.

TREATMENT OF INDIGESTION, WITH ILLUSTRATIVE CASES.

1. *Improper Food.*

CASE I.—CONVULSIONS FROM EATING INDIGESTIBLE FOOD, CURED BY *Nux vomica*.

SOME years ago I was called in a great hurry to see a girl, about eight years old, in convulsions. The child was completely unconscious, was struggling violently, the eyes were distorted, and the face dark. It was the beginning of the fruit season, and I discovered that she had eaten some foreign plums an hour or so before the attack came on. There was scarcely any remission in the convulsions; she went out of one into another. I mixed a few drops of *Nux vomica* in water, and put a little of it between her teeth every two or three minutes. After a few doses she was quieter, and at last was able to swallow the medicine. I stayed with her for about an hour, by which time the convulsions had entirely ceased, and they did not return. She passed a quantity of the indigestible fruit by the bowels, and the next day was quite well.

Nux vomica is the most frequently called for remedy in cases of acute indigestion from improper food. But if the food is of a rich or fat kind, as fat pork, *Pulsatilla* must be given.

The dieting in these cases is a simple affair. No food of any kind should be given until the attack is over. If there is thirst, water or toast-water may be given, as much as is desired.

When habitual disregard of the

stomach's requirements has set up a chronic indigestion, the same remedies will be demanded according to their symptoms. Consult also in the MATERIA MEDICA, *Arsen.*, *Hydrast.*, *Ac. carbol.*, *Kali bichrom.*, and the chapter on DIET.

2. *Irregularities of Diet.*

CASE II.—EXTREME DYSPEPSIA WITH MENTAL SYMPTOMS FROM IRREGULARITIES OF DIET, ETC.,—*Sulphur*, *Lycopodium*, and *Nux vomica*.

In November, 1890, I was written to from the country by a young lady complaining of inability to take any kind of food, more especially meat, without the most intense suffering, bodily and mental. From her description of her case I gathered that she might be helped by treatment, and asked her to come to town to see me, which she did, accompanied by a friend. She was extremely thin, somewhat anæmic, with the ruddy complexion on a pale skin that is found in many cases of anæmia. She looked greatly depressed, and was, in fact, in very low spirits; very irritable, and liked to be alone.

Up to the previous June she had been in excellent health. In that month she had visited a sister who was ill, and helped to nurse her. This entailed much worry, and she was subjected to *great irregularity in the times of taking meals.* In addition to this she was frequently exposed to cold, going out in thin shoes and getting her feet wet when heated.

The first symptoms which ensued were —continual and almost unbearable pains in the back, severe headaches, loss of appetite, and unpleasant taste in the mouth, and a great distaste for meat. She had great thirst, and the bowels were constipated. At last she could not take the smallest piece of anything without great pain, and she became dreadfully low-spirited and cried much. She had a "queer feeling in her head as if she could not think." She took medical advice, but did not improve. In August her friends became so much alarmed about her condition, both mental and bodily, that they induced her to go away for a change to the seaside. There things got worse rather than better. She forced herself to eat in spite of the intense pain and general discomfort the food caused; she had constant nausea, especially in the morning, and either had diarrhœa or was constipated. Returning home she tried starving herself, taking only liquid foods and not much of them, and she found that the less she took of anything the better she felt, though she became very weak and felt dreadfully exhausted at times.

Things went on very much in this way till she consulted me in November.

Her condition at that time was as follows:—

She was extremely thin and weak. Though quite young, her hair was grayish, and had been so for three months. Her face burned frequently, and more especially after food. Her tongue was white; she had thick white phlegm in the throat, which felt sore and rough in the evening.

The especial dyspeptic symptoms were the following,—a craving for food and a sense of weight felt in the lowest part of the abdomen, and made worse by eating. Sinking, empty feeling all day. Flatulence both of stomach and bowels. Vomits food at times. Sour eructations at times, and sometimes she hawks or coughs up white or yellow phlegm. Rumbling in the bowels, distension after food, particularly after breakfast. Bowels always constipated; motions dark, accompanied with pain; urine has been very thick and red, with sediment at times.

There was aching in chest in the morning on waking. Pulse slow and soft. Continual and almost unbearable pain in the back. Aching in limbs from exertion. Feet very cold; hands and feet used formerly to perspire much, but have not done so for the last three or four months. Sleep poor, wakes between 3 and 4 A. M. She is very chilly, and is better when warm. She received *Sulphur* as a medicine, and was told that in spite of the suffering it gave her she must persevere in taking food. She was to have scalded milk (that is, cold milk into which an equal quantity of boiling water has been poured) in place of tea and coffee. Breakfast at 8, of porridge, raw egg or bacon. At 1 o'clock, beef-tea, milk pudding, no vegetables. At 5, toast with scalded milk. At 8.30, bread and milk.

In a fortnight she reported herself better in some respects. The pain in the back was less severe. She had not vomited, though the nausea continued. She complained of a sensation as if the food rose up into the throat and stuck there. There was less flatulence. The urine was clearer. The bowels were still confined, though she had an action each day. She felt the intense cold of the weather very much. She still slept badly. Eggs disagreed with her.

The next prescription was *Lycopodium;* and in the way of diet I ordered Nichol's "Food of Health" (a preparation of wheat) in place of oatmeal porridge. The *Lycopodium* seemed to aggravate her symptoms; she felt less well; the constipation became worse; she had a worrying headache in forehead and left temple; thick jelly-like and greenish or yellow phlegm from upper part of throat came after eating. The *Lycopodium* was now replaced by *Nux vomica,* and this made a speedy change for the better. In a week the pains in the body and back were much better; the headaches had gone; the constipation was better; she could eat eggs without any discomfort; and her spirits were very much better. Though still waking early in the morning, she was practically quite well in body and mind by the end of January. I forgot to mention, as showing the alarming state she was in, that the friend who came with her when she visited me first, asked me privately, after the interview, if I did not think the patient was going out of her mind. My reply was, that the mental condition was secondary to the bodily disease, and would become all right when the latter was remedied.

This was a case in which the condition had gone so far that mere reform in diet was not sufficient to restore the patient; the additional help of the gentle powers of homœopathic medicines was needed for the cure.

3. *Alcohol.*

The value of *Nux vomica* in dissipating the effects of a too free indulgence in the pleasures of the table is too well known to need illustrating. The splitting headache, dirty tongue, and absence of appetite, experienced the following morning, sends the delinquent who has once tried it to the *Nux vomica* bottle ever after. Older sinners, with tremulous, white-coated tongue, vomiting in the morning, pale face, and no appetite, will find some relief from *Antim. tart.*, and if they can be persuaded to give up their tippling habits, they may recover and preserve a measure of the strength they have squandered.

And even when it has come to a case of "hob-nail" liver and dropsy, hope must not be abandoned, as the following case will show :—

CASE III.—CHRONIC ALCOHOLISM ; CIRRHOSIS OF THE LIVER; DROPSY; INDIGESTION ; GREAT AMELIORATION, —*China*, *Kali carb.*

On the 11th of December, 1886, there came to my clinique at the Homœopathic Hospital a man, E. T., aged 45, an inspector on the railway by occupation. He was a tall, large man, having his face covered with the red spots characteristic of spirit drinkers. He had recently been discharged from St Thomas's Hospital as incurable, having been in there thirteen weeks, during which period he was tapped four times for dropsy. Ever since he was tapped the third time he had suffered from pain about the navel shortly after anything he had eaten or drunk.

In addition to this, he complained of swelling of the limbs and body, coldness of the hands, pain in the bowels, the motions being light, and bad sleep. The tongue was clean, the appetite good in spite of the pain caused by eating. There was much dropsy of the legs and body, the liver was hard and small, and its sharp edge could be distinctly felt beneath the ribs. He had been a great drinker, his favourite drink being gin and water, cold. When he left St. Thomas's Hospital he was not warned about his drinking habits.

Nine months previous to the date of my seeing him first, he had been for six weeks under his club doctor, and received so much benefit that he thought he was cured.

Three years previously he had lost his wife and his health had never been the same after. He suffered from rheumatic gout at times. Sixteen years before, he had gastric fever very badly, but except for these had never suffered from any illness.

When this patient came to me first I happened to have several medical students connected with St. Thomas's Hospital watching my work, and as they were acquainted with the case of E. T., and the treatment he had received at St. Thomas's, and its results, they were anxious to see what else could be done for him.

I prescribed *China* in the 1^x dilution to be taken three times a day, with the same medicine in the 30th dilution to be taken at bedtime. I also cautioned him about his drinking habits, but I regret to say, without very much effect.

He returned in a fortnight, and his former hospital acquaintances were able to note a marked change for the better,

He had lost all pains after food, and also the pains in his limbs, which were smaller; the abdomen was less distended; the motions were darker in colour, and a troublesome cough from which he suffered was better also.

Under this same medicine he steadily improved ; gradually all the dropsy disappeared out of his legs, and he was able to do his work with comfort. Once, when his face became very troublesome, the pimples being inflamed and red, I gave him *Kali carb.* 30 for a few days, and with good effect. This was the only alteration I made in the original prescription, and he ceased attending on March 25th.

He continued at work till the following autumn, and might have been at work still, in my opinion, if he could only have kept from alcohol. This, however, he failed to do, and I heard that he died after a very short illness following a severe cold.

4. *Tobacco.*

CASE IV. — AGGRAVATED DYSPEPSIA CAUSED BY TOBACCO POISONING, CURED MAINLY BY *Nux vomica.*

At Christmas, 1886, an active man of business came up from the country to place himself under my care with symptoms of acute indigestion. He was 46 years of age, short but stout, and had been exceedingly strong; his complexion was dark and rather sallow. There was not much doubt about the cause of his indigestion. He had commenced to smoke at 12, and had continued to use the drug in excess, both chewing and smoking, until a year before he came to see me. At that time he had met with an accident, being thrown from his trap, and after this his health failed rapidly. He began to be sick after his breakfast; had tingling in his right thigh; lost flesh; was bilious and depressed. He left off his after-breakfast pipe, and only smoked after his dinner. The sickness then ceased for a time, but soon returned as badly as ever. He consulted several medical men, and received a little help from some of them. In September a lay friend, who is skillful in the use of Homœopathy, happening to be visiting at his house, took him in hand, and gave him *Nux vomica.* At that time smoking was an impossibility; he vomited as soon as he attempted to smoke; his sickness was extreme; he could not walk along the street without vomiting. Under *Nux vomica* he improved in a surprising manner, and soon regained appetite and digestion. In a week he felt so well that he thought he might try a pipe again. Again the sickness came on as violently as before, and this time, though the *Nux* helped him, it did not restore him so completely as at first. Now his sensitiveness to tobacco was so great that he could not bear to be in a room where anyone was smoking.

When he came under my care, *Nux* was again the chief agent in his restoration. *Calc. carb.* was very efficient in correcting the acidity which was one of his symptoms, and *Iodide of Arsenic* also did him great good, but *Nux* again practically cured him. He was able, when I heard from him last, to eat any kind of food ; he attended to his business, and was steadily gaining weight. Of course all this time he abstained from tobacco.

Besides the remedies used in this case, *Ipecac.* is also a useful remedy in tobacco dyspepsia, relieving the sickness greatly.

CASE V.—INDIGESTION WITH INDURATED LIVER; ALCOHOLIC HISTORY.

A city gentleman, about 50, came to me in the summer of 1895, complaining of a pain in his left flank and round the body, giddiness, flatulence, and great depression of spirits. Eight years before he had had stone in the bladder. For the last two or three years he had suffered from liver symptoms, and since then he had been very chilly, whereas previously he never felt the cold. He had had eczema severely, but he found out that it was only when he took fruit. The giddiness occurred when he turned his head. This had troubled him at times since the previous winter, when he had several severe attacks, the first one occurring in a train.

His tongue was dirty. Good appetite except for breakfast. His appetite was better than his digestion. Formerly he had been in the habit of drinking too much beer, but recently he had taken none, though he had not given up alcohol altogether. He had a sinking sensation at the epigastrium before lunch. Had a pain in left flank and all round the abdomen *when he moved.* The bowels used to be constipated, but since he had taken *Carbo veg.* on his own account that had been remedied, and he had discarded the use of Hunyadi Janos water, on which he had depended before. He had a pain in the soft part of the loins going round to the front on both sides. The fingers were shrivelled as in cholera patients; and after washing there was a peculiar odour from the tips, lasting a long time.

On examination I found his liver was considerably enlarged, and very hard and tender. There was a venous zig-zag along the attachment of the diaphragm. The indication for *Bryonia*, especially the marked aggravation from movement, was sufficiently clear, and he received that medicine in the 30th.

Sixteen days later he reported that the pain gradually disappeared, also the deadness of the fingers; was free from headache, but had slept badly on account of irritation at the rectum.

℞. *Sul.* 30 ter die. *Verbascum* Ointment.

Three weeks later he reported himself much better. Irritation gone. Very little indigestion. The liver was softer, though the spleen dulness was increased. He was suffering from a cold, for which *Cepa* 30 was given with relief, and then he had *Nat. mur.* 30. *Calc. c.* and *Psor.* 30 were given later, and he lost all his distressing symptoms, though his weight remained much below his normal.

CASE VI.—TOBACCO AND WHISKY DYSPEPSIA—*Lycopodium*.

Here is a somewhat similar case of more recent date. J. M., 35, wrote to me from the north of Scotland in May, 1890, complaining of indigestion which had troubled him for four years, before which time he had been exceptionally strong.

The chief symptoms he complained of

were: A sweetish taste in the mouth; tongue thickly coated, white in the morning and yellow in the evening; hot, burninig risings in the throat, which was inflamed at the right side sometimes; white sediment in the urine after standing. Besides these he had other related symptoms; he was unable to think at times, could not concentrate his thoughts on any matter he had to do, and at those times he had a feeling as if the blood were running cold in his head; he was either very drowsy or sleepy, or else very cross, and his sleep was unrefreshing. He was always chilly, always catching cold, and obliged to wear very heavy clothing. He was a heavy smoker, and also took whisky. These I stopped, and also forbade all kinds of stimulating food and drinks. The medicine I prescribed was *Nux vom.* in a high attenuation.

In a month he wrote that he was still troubled a good deal with the sour risings, the condition of the mouth, and the white sediment in the urine. It was evident the *Nux* was not a sufficiently deeply-acting remedy to reach his complaint; though for the purpose of antidoting the effect of his bad habits and of preparing the way for the constitutional remedy, it was the natural one to think of first. The next medicine on the list of similars was *Lycopodium*, the leading indications being—acid risings, sore throat, worse on right side, white sediment in urine (though with *Lycopodium* it is more characteristically *red*), excessive chilliness, mental confusion. I sent him three powders of the medicine in the same attenuation, with directions to take one at bedtime, one the following morning, and one again at bedtime. The medicine was now allowed to act without further repetition.

The change wrought by these three doses may be estimated by the man's own words. Writing a month later, he said,

"I have felt much better with the last medicine than the first. The tongue is less white, sometimes the coat has cleaned right off, though it has come on again. I feel much stronger now and *quite warm.*" No more medicine was given or required. The increase in the bodily heat is a sure sign of regained vitality.

5. *Tea.*

CASE VII.—TEA DYSPEPSIA, CURED BY *Merc. sol.*, *Actæa racemosa*, *etc.*

Emma E., 39, dressmaker, consulted me at the London Homœopathic Hospital on June 21st, 1883, complaining of the following symptoms:—Great nervousness; pain in the left side when she ate; sensation as if there was a weight on the shoulders and back, especially when tired; aching in the nape of the neck all day; offensive breath, bleeding gums, bad taste in the mouth, white tongue; restless sleep. The bowels were regular and the appetite good. She took her meals at regular times, and drank *nine* cups of tea in a day.

I told her she must give up her tea, and gave her *Merc. sol.* 6, in drop doses four times a day.

She returned in a fortnight, and reported that she had reduced her allowance to *six* cups daily.

The sharp pains she complained of were better than they had been for years, and she slept better; the breath was still offensive. Repeat medicine.

She was not able to attend for a few weeks, and having been out of medicine was not so well. She was so very nervous. By this time she had got down to *four* cups a day. Repeat medicine.

On Aug. 11th, she received *Act. rac.* for headache, and did not return till Oct. 6th, when she reported that the medicine had done her head good, but now she had soreness of the chest, and much flatulence. *Carbo veg.* 6, one drop four times a day.

Nov. 3.—Has kept well till to-day. Now has palpitation ; headache at the back of the head ; sore feeling within the head ; giddiness ; flatulence. *Gels.* 1, one drop four times a day.

On Nov. 17, a fortnight after, she reported that she had not been so well for years. The head was very much better, and she had hardly any of the palpitation. She had now brought herself to *two* cups of tea a day. She received more of the medicine, and soon after ceased to attend.

In each instance the medicine given responded admirably to its indications, but I question if she would have received much benefit if she had not, besides, cut down her allowance of tea. It is possible to antidote a poison when the poison is being taken, but it is easier to antidote its effects when it is no longer present. Sometimes the effects of a poison, if not antidoted, will last for years after the last dose has been taken.

CASE VIII.—TEA DYSPEPSIA.

The next case I give not as an example of treatment, but as a typical case of the disease. The patient, for some reason or other, did not persevere with the treatment, but she has left me her history, and here I give it—

M. G., 42, housewife, presented herself at the Homœopathic Hospital on Sept. 8th, 1883.

She complained of pain in the chest, which she had had for weeks ; bad sleep ; pressure on the chest on falling asleep ; white tongue ; poor appetite ; headache across the forehead. She drank much tea, taking it three or four times a day.

She felt very ill after it, especially if she took it hot.

Bryonia made no improvement in her case; she had much sickness and retching, and the head was very sore. She did not report herself after the second visit.

Tea produces two sets of symptoms, nervous and dyspeptic, and sometimes both combined. In some it produces fits of low spirits, and no other disorder. When taken to great excess, it causes paralysis. Besides the medicines given in the above reported cases, *China*, *Ferrum*, *Thuja*, and *Arsenic* are good antidotes to tea poisoning.

6. *Arsenic.*

CASE IX.—ARSENIC DYSPEPSIA, CURED BY *Bryonia*.

Speaking of *Arsenic* reminds me of a frequent cause of dyspepsia, which I have not particularly specified in the preceding chapter, but which I will illustrate here.

A young married woman came to me some time ago, complaining of symptoms of dyspepsia, chiefly weight at the stomach and pains through from the pit of the stomach to the back between the shoulders after everything she ate. She was pale and her lips were somewhat pallid. The tongue was red, with a white silvery coating; the bowels were confined. She was temperate in all her habits.

I suspected *Arsenic* at once. She said that her husband suffered from similar symptoms, and I told her to bring me some of her wall-paper, giving her *Bryonia* to take until she came next. When she returned she reported very great improvement in the symptoms. This might have made me doubt my first diagnosis, did I not know that it is possible to cure an effect sometimes even whilst the cause remains. I examined the paper, and then found *Arsenic* in great quantity. When the paper was taken away, both she and her husband became perfectly well.

7. *Cold.*

CASE X.—DYSPEPSIA FROM COLD, CURED BY *Carbo veg.*

Exposure to cold has the effect of stopping digestion, the result of which is, in a general way, to produce a great quantity of gas in the stomach and intestines.

A professional man, riding home on the top of an omnibus, facing a cold wind, felt pains in his chest and body of a sharp cutting kind. He had experienced the same thing on previous occasions, and had at times suffered off and on for days from weak digestion, the symptoms returning after every meal. On this particular occasion, a few drops of *Carbo veg.* 6 relieved him at once of all his trouble.

CASE XI.—DYSPEPSIA FROM COLD—*Plumbum.*

A young lady, after leaving off a flannel skirt for some obscure reason in cold weather, was seized with violent pains in her body, aggravated after everything she ate, no matter what. The pains kept her awake at night, and she had cramp in her calves and constipation. After some remedies had been given without benefit, *Plumbum* 6 cured her on this occasion, and also subsequently when a similar imprudence brought on a renewal of the attack.

8. *Bad Air.*

CASE XII.—DYSPEPSIA FROM BAD AIR.

Wm. D., 33, lithographer, consulted me at the Homœopathic Hospital for indigestion, flatulence, inability to sleep, loss of memory, and constipation. He was temperate and did not smoke. He worked much over gas, and to this I attribute the greater part of the symptoms. *Nux vomica* made a great alteration for the better in all his symptoms, and he did not return till two months later. Then he had a return of the old symptoms with piles, and again *Nux*, with a dose of *Sulphur* at bedtime, put him right.

9. *Vinegar Dyspepsia.*

When acidity and flatulence are the leading symptoms of this form of dyspepsia, *Carbo veg.* is the best remedy. When the wasting is extreme, *Iodine* must be given.

10. *Tight-lacing Dyspepsia.*

The symptoms of this kind of dyspepsia are very varied, and will call for a great variety of rèmedies. Of course, the chief remedy is to discard stays and let the ribs have their natural motion, and the abdominal organs room to act properly. *Nux vomica*, *Carbo veg.*, *Bryonia*, *Ignatia*, and *Sulphur*, must be consulted.

11. *Dyspepsia from Nervous Debility.*

CASE XIII.—DYSPEPSIA FROM NERVOUS SHOCK—*Iodine.*

A young lady of gouty family, but enjoying good health, active, well nourished, and somewhat stout, met with a severe nervous shock. From that time her health failed. She lost appetite, all food becoming distasteful to her, she had frequent attacks of vomiting, and from being stout, wasted rapidly. She had been under treatment before coming to me, and had received some benefit, but not much. After trying one or two medicines, I put her on *Iodine*, and on this she began to recover steadily. After taking this some time she was restored to a large measure of health and comfort, though when she left off treatment she was not quite the same as she was before the shock.

This is one type of dyspepsia from nervous weakness. Business causes and continued anxieties are equally prejudicial to digestion, and are best removed by such medicines as *Ignatia*.

But there is another and often more serious kind of dyspepsia, where the disease is due not to mental but to physical causes. The usual history is the acquirement of evil habits at school, young boys being led on by those older and wickeder than themselves. These habits are indulged in secretly, until something happens to startle the youth into a sense of his criminal folly.

CASE XIV.—DYSPEPSIA RESULTING FROM NERVOUS DEBILITY.

A youth with the above history consulted me a year or so ago for his indigestion. He had great flatulence, which he was continually belching, acidity, and heartburn, great sleepiness (which was a serious trouble to him, as he was working for an examination). He had queer feelings in his head, and had attacks of nausea, but did not vomit. His bowels were constipated. He came of a dyspeptic family, and had been allowed to eat indigestible things when a child, but that was not the cause of his present attack, though both circumstances helped to make it the difficult case it was to treat.

There were certain things that made his symptoms worse. The eructations were worse after eating water-melon or rice pudding, and much worse after blanc-mange and custard.

He had a voracious appetite.

I put him on a very strict regimen, which he faithfully followed. He had been in the habit of dining in the middle of the day, and taking tea in the afternoon about four hours after his dinner, and a supper late.

I told him to take only three meals a day, at 8:30, 1 and 6:30. He was never to eat as much as he could; he was to take no tea nor stimulants of any kind, but to drink for breakfast, milk with boiling water, take only a very light meal in the middle of the day, of beef or mutton, vegetables (excluding potatoes), and some milk pudding; a similar meal was to be taken at 6:30, and nothing after or between. For breakfast I allowed him bacon with stale bread, toast or biscuit. After the last meal he was not to study, but to read light things, and take a two miles' walk before going to bed.

Then I cut down his sleeping hours. He had been sleeping too much, from about 10:30 to 7:30. I ordered him to be in bed at 10:45, and to rise at 6:45, take a cold sponge bath and work before breakfast.

Under this regimen he made considerable improvement, but the chief features of his indigestion remained unchanged.

Nux vom. gave him a great deal of help, and *Nux moschata* did something towards relieving the drowsiness. *Acid. phos.* 1_x, five drops in water for a beverage, to be drunk at lunch and dinner, also proved helpful. *Calc. c.* and *Puls.* relieved the acidity, and finally *Natrum muriaticum* completed the cure, relieving constipation as well as the other remaining symptoms of indigestion.

He was altogether under treatment about 10 months. At the end of this time he was able to work many hours a day without feeling any drowsiness. He could eat eggs, rice and other articles without inconvenience; and he was able to make a good appearance in a scholarship examination.

I have found *Nat. mur.* of immense service in similar cases. *China*, *Ignatia*, *Platina*, *Oxalic acid*, and *Sulphur* have also helped much.

12. *Indigestion and Chlorosis.*

Anæmia, green-sickness, or chlorosis is attended with indigestion as one of its main symptoms.

CASE XV.—INDIGESTION OF CHLOROSIS CURED BY *Petroleum*.

Not long ago I was asked to see the maid of a patient of mine. She was pale and bloodless to an intense degree, had no appetite, loathed meat, and could hardly be persuaded to swallow solid food of any kind. It gave her pain and made her sick. She had great breathlessness on exertion, especially on going upstairs, of which she had much to do in the course of the day. I put her on milk diet, and allowed her nothing else. At first she was only able to take this diluted with boiling water. This effected some improvement. I then gave her as a medicine *Petroleum*, and the benefit was soon manifest. The sickness left her; she was able to take other food besides milk, and with appetite; her colour came back, and the catamenia, which had completely stopped, returned. She was able to do her work with much less difficulty, for she did not give up for a single day.

Here is a similar case:—

CASE XVI.—DYSPEPSIA OF ANÆMIA SIMULATING ULCERATION OF THE STOMACH CURED BY *Argent. nit.*

Alice C., 15, consulted me at the Homœopathic Hospital. She complained of severe pain after eating. It had been worse the last three weeks. She had had the same pain the previous winter. The pain was in the pit of the stomach, which was very tender. It came on an hour after food. She grew sick, but did not vomit. She was thirsty and had no appetite. The tongue was clean; bowels regular. She had had diarrhœa.

The pulse was frequent; she was very breathless; was pale, and had all the symptoms of anæmia.

I gave her *Argentum nitricum* thrice daily, and all the indigestion symptoms disappeared. She told me that when she had missed taking the medicine at proper times, she had had return of the pain.

In this case there was more pain and less sickness and absence of appetite than in the one cured by *Petroleum*. Also the anæmia was less intense.

13. *Drug Dyspepsia.*

When dyspepsia is the result of frequent drugging, the first thing to do is to stop everything in the shape of drugs, and put the patient on strict rules of diet. He should not be closely restricted to *articles* of diet, but should be very particular about the *time* of feeding, giving the stomach proper intervals of rest. He must beware of taking too little food. Dyspeptics of this kind are very apt to leave off by degrees one article of diet after another which they have found disagrees with them (and everything disagrees), till they have hardly anything left that they can eat. They must be encouraged to be a little daring, and as everything will give them pain at first, to eat everything except the most indigestible articles. In this way the stomach will become accustomed much more to proper meals. When this treatment has been pursued for some time, then Homœopathy will be able to step in and help the patient. In these cases there is no very definite set of symptoms, and therefore the *Materia Medica* must be consulted to discern which drug is likeliest in its effect to the condition of the patient.

14. *Miscellaneous Kinds.*

Among the unclassed kinds of dyspepsia I will mention next the case of a young lady who was never well in London, and never ill out of it.

CASE XVII.—LONDON DYSPEPSIA—*Abies nigra.*

This patient had been under me some years before for a sharp attack of inflammation of the bowels, recovery from which was greatly retarded by an arsenical wall paper with which her bed-room was papered.

Now, whenever she is in London she has violent attacks of indigestion, and also has constipation. The pain she suffers is in the pit of the stomach, and right side. It is of a cramping, tearing nature, and is much worse when the bowels are relieved. She has great chilliness. She cannot eat meat or any solid food, and is obliged to restrict herself to a diet of milk with boiling water (in place of tea or coffee), revalenta, figs stewed in milk, and biscuits in place of bread. I found some medicines help her a little, especially *Abies nigra*, which relieved the pain, the chilliness, and the constipation, and seemed at one time as if it was going to cure her. But the constipation returned, though not the dyspeptic symptoms in their old intensity. However, nothing cured her till she went into the country, and within a week of her leaving she was able to eat anything she liked, and the bowels gave no trouble at all.

I have known the reverse of this happen—people who are healthy in London and yet suffer all kinds of discomfort when living at home in the midst of a pine-forest.

CASE XVIII. — DYSPEPSIA OF SIX YEARS' STANDING CURED BY *Abies*.

A barrister consulted me in the autumn of 1886 about an indigestion from which he had suffered for six years. He was temperate, and there was no clear cause for his trouble. His symptoms were oppression, feeling as if something stuck in the pit of his stomach, flatulence, tendency to constipation, depression, great chilliness, difficulty in concentrating his thoughts; he felt worse when he ate a good deal. His pulse was 84, soft. Before his illness came on he had had exceedingly good health. The symptoms all pointed to one medicine, *Abies nigra*. I gave this, and the one prescription practically cured him. When he returned, though his symptoms had not all gone, he was practically a different creature. The pain at the stomach pit had almost disappeared. He was no longer chilly. He was able to work better. His bowels were open. I repeated his medicine, and that completed the cure.

15. *Constitutional Indigestion.*

When indigestion is one of the symptoms of a morbid constitutional state—whether gout or rheumatism, or one of those designated by Hahnemann *psora* and *sycosis*—the treatment will have to be adapted to the constitution, and not directed to the stomach alone or chiefly, as when that organ is primarily at fault.

The remedies most useful in dyspepsia of gout are, *Sulphur*, *Carbo vegetabilis*, and *Lycopodium*. Patients who have loss of appetite every spring and autumn, and find they cannot digest eggs as they can at other times, who suffer from drowsiness, heaviness on waking, unpleasant taste in the mouth, and possibly constipation, will be greatly benefited by a few doses of *Sulphur.* Others who have flatulence with pains in the chest, are chilly, and yet desire air; bowels open or loose, require *Carbo veg. Lycopodium* is suited for those who have flatulence in the bowels, with constipation, and urine giving a red deposit.

I will now relate two cases in point.

CASE XIX.—A CHRONIC CONSTITUTIONAL CASE WITH DILATED STOMACH; RECURRENT FISTULA, CURED WITH *Sulphur.*

A year or two back an officer in the army, who had seen a good deal of service abroad, came to consult me about his digestion. He was 45 years of age, and though a man of large frame, was wasted to a degree. He brought with him a photograph taken before the illness commenced, and it was difficult to recognize any resemblance between it and the patient in his then condition.

His history in brief was as follows :— For ten years he had had indigestion with constipation and piles. He had lost much flesh, especially in the last year. In India he had had fever and had taken much quinine. Lately he had taken much quack medicine, principally for opening the bowels.

Seventeen years before I saw him he had had a "boil" form near the anus, and ever since then after great exertion he had had a recurrence of anal abscess and fistula. The last time was eight months before. It bled much, but had never formed again, and since that time his indigestion had been worse. He had been a great smoker, but for ten months had not smoked at all.

When he came to me he was having attacks every week of violent vomiting. In two minutes he would vomit as much as a gallon of fluid, sour or sweet. The least exertion caused him to vomit. There was pain and great thirst in the stomach, but not severe. The stomach I found to be considerably dilated, the spleen somewhat enlarged, and there were some enlarged glands in the groin.

The tongue was dirty; often there was a bad taste, and the mouth was clammy and sticky in the morning. Up till ten years before, the bowels had been regular, but since then has had constipation, which he has taken purgatives to relieve. The piles were not painful, but bled, and at times came down. He had cramp in the calves, and cold, dry feet. Sleep was restless. He took long to go off, and waked early in the morning. He was very irritable and wished to be left alone.

I gave him *Sulphur* 30 three times a

day, and told him to take no purgatives, but to use enemata if necessary.

In a month he reported himself very much better, and it was plain to see that he was quite a different man. He had had much fewer attacks, and those that came were less severe. He had been able to eat meat again without discomfort, though he had been subsisting on porridge and gruel chiefly before. The excessive thirst had gone, and though the constipation remained, the piles were very much better. The urine, which had been thick and offensive, was now normal. Sleeps better, though he still wakes at 4 A.M. *Sulphur* 30 twice a day, and *Nux v.* at bedtime.

In another month still further improvement was apparent. He had filled out to such an extent that he did not at all belie his photograph. He complained chiefly of his appetite being too good, being most hungry in the afternoons. At times the thirst returned, and he had flatulence sometimes. There was still a tendency to early waking.

Lycopodium was now given, and that completed the cure.

Now this was a decidedly constitutional case. The indigestion was only one manifestation of his ailment, and this became worse when the fistula healed. The fistula and the indigestion were not two complaints—but one; and only deeply acting constitutional remedies, homœopathically related to all affected parts of the organism could have cured the patient. Severe measures, such as surgical treatment of the piles, or acids or alkalies to correct the state of the stomach, though sanctified by the approval of the highest scientific authority in the old school, is the merest cobbling work, and no true cure at all.

CASE XX.—A CHRONIC CASE ARISING FROM AN IMPROPERLY TREATED SKIN AFFECTION. *Sulphur, Nux moschata.*

This patient was a clerk in the city in the early twenties, and he complained of having had indigestion twelve months. It came on suddenly one day after taking tea, and he could not account for it in any way. His principal symptom was that his food lay like a weight at the umbilical region. Sour eructations, and rising into the throat of bits of the last food taken. Bad taste in the mouth at times; good appetite; takes rather much salt. Thirsty after dinner, which he takes in the evening, and which is the meal which gives most trouble. Spirits low; headache occasionally. Sleepy after meals. Prefers cold weather, but always feels cold and is sensitive to draughts. Is a total abstainer and a non-smoker.

Sulph. 30 ter die.

A fortnight later he reported himself as

much better, and for several weeks under *Puls.*, *Lyc.*, and *Sulph.* the improvement went on with fluctuations.

One day he mentioned, among other symptoms, that his saliva was very thick, like cotton.

℞ *Nux mosch.* 30 ter die for a week, to be followed with *Sulph.* 30 for the next week.

Whilst taking the *Nux moschata* the symptoms of indigestion vanished; but, to quote his own words, "singularly enough, the same eruption appeared as existed before I had the indigestion." The *Sulph.* rather sent matters back this time, so I gave *Nux mosch.* again.

I now for the first time obtained the history of the eruption.

It was one of acne, which had been "cured" by local applications. In other words, the complaint had been driven from his skin to his internal organs.

He was subject to eruptions when young. Shaving was now difficult, the skin being so tender. *Carbo an* put that right. The *Nux moschata* made him less chilly, and he did not require much medicine after these had done their work.

Rheumatic dyspepsia will find its specifics in *Bryonia*, *Kali bichromicum* (especially where rheumatic pains and dyspeptic symptoms alternate), or *Sulphur*. The *psoric* individual will require very careful treating. The medicine of the widest range in the treatment of these cases is *Sulphur*, but his symptoms will require close study and accurate comparison with the symptoms of the drugs in order to find the drug that most closely corresponds. For the hydrogenoid or sycotic constitution, in which the patient suffers intermittently from indigestion, with other symptoms, worse on every change of the weather, and especially when the air is damp and cold, *Arsen.*, *Nux*, *Ipec.*, and *Natrum mur.* will be found most useful according to the indications given in the *Materia Medica*.

CHAPTER VI.

DIET IN DYSPEPSIA.

IT is just as easy to give too little food to dyspeptics as too much. When a stomach has once become whimsical, its whims will have to be disregarded in the process of breaking it into more wholesome habits. Of course, this will mean a certain amount of suffering at first, but the good results of it will soon be apparent.

When there is ulceration of the stomach present, it will be necessary to give only liquid food, and of all liquid foods in these states, koumiss is the best.

In acute attacks of indigestion the best of all remedies is to go without any food at all until the stomach has had time to recover itself.

In the chronic cases where the vitality is low, and the general tone of health not robust, great care will be required in bringing the patient back to ordinary diet. Cold foods must be particularly avoided. Bread only sparingly used. Bread is not nearly so digestible an article as most people imagine, and dyspeptics should never eat bread and butter, or hot buttered toast. Dry toast is all they should indulge in. When toast is not tolerated, rusks or biscuits may take its place. Plain water-biscuits are the best;

such as Huntly & Palmer's "Breakfast biscuits," and "Captain's biscuits;" Cracknell's; and Spiking's (Dover Street, Piccadilly) "Oval Cheese biscuits," and "Lunch biscuits." For breakfast there is one cold article of diet dyspeptics may take, and that is the fat of very good cold boiled bacon. They may have this with toast.

Tea is bad for the digestion, and the habit of drinking tea in the afternoon is an exceedingly objectionable one. It breaks up the proper interval between lunch and dinner, and gives the tea its best possible chance of working its evil effects on the stomach. Coffee is not so injurious to the digestion as tea. It rather assists the digestion of fats which tea hinders. Though coffee has more tendency to cause headache, and with some persons flatulence and constipation, with others it assists the action of the bowels. Tea should never be taken without milk or cream, and it should never be strong, or taken after it has been made more than a few minutes.

The teas of China are less injurious than those of India and Ceylon. Green teas are especially poisonous, and should never be taken under any circumstances.

Cocoa possesses more of the nutrient and sustaining properties, and is less of a pure stimulant than either tea or coffee. Some object to it on that account, as they say they want a drink rather than a food. This difficulty may be avoided by using some of the lighter forms of cocoa, as Epps' Cocoaine, an extract made from the nibs; or the nibs themselves, or the shells may be used for making the beverage.

When meat cannot be taken, beef-tea must be substituted. Mutton is more digestible than beef, because in beef the fat is more intermixed with the fibre of the meat, and the fat is more difficult to digest, and the fibre is harder.

In cases where there is manifest ulceration of the stomach, koumiss is the best food. It may be given alone every hour or every two hours, until the pain and vomiting have ceased and other food can be taken. When koumiss is not obtainable, milk and lime-water, or milk and soda-water may be substituted.

When dyspepsia is constitutional the particular constitution must be studied.

Gouty patients should avoid all rich or highly-spiced foods, and eat little butter and milk except with tea or coffee. These should be taken not strong, and the tea only when freshly made. Meat should be taken once a day, never cold, and never cooked a second time. The less flatulent kinds of vegetables are good, as French beans, spinach, young peas, also stewed celery. Potatoes should be avoided, and cabbage. Malt liquors, wines, and spirits should be avoided. Water is the best drink at meals; Salutaris water or toast water may be substituted. Hard water should be carefully avoided. Gouty patients should drink freely of liquids.

Those who have a tendency to rheumatism should observe most of the rules indicated for the gouty. Excess of meat and milk are not good. Oatmeal porridge should be taken at breakfast; at lunch or dinner, soup, meat from the joint, with vegetables, plain rice or other farinaceous pudding without eggs, and no fruit. Toast-water should be the drink with the meals. Fresh-water fish, and watery fruits and vegetables, must be avoided.

For the psoric no special rules

can be laid down. They must be dieted according to their symptoms. The chilly "*sycotic*" patients must avoid all cold foods and watery foods, as the rheumatic. They may drink hot water, but never cold water. It will often be found beneficial to the circulation to sponge them every morning all over with spirit of wine before dressing. Fruit, milk, melons, mushrooms, hard-boiled eggs must be avoided.

Oysters can sometimes be taken when nothing else can, and they contain a considerable amount of nourishment. They may be taken raw or cooked as desired.

Pepsine and all the artificial digestives I do not like, except for short periods. The stomach is ready enough to accommodate itself to inaction; and when it finds the food put into it already peptonised, it will not trouble itself to secrete any pepsine itself. Hence it falls into bad habits, and finally the artificial pepsine ceases to suit the patient, whose stomach is then really weaker than before the pepsine was given.

An exception must be made in favour of a preparation I have found very useful, namely, *Bullock's Acid Glycerine of Pepsine*, a teaspoonful being mixed in half a tumbler of hot water, and drunk at meals as a beverage. This is very pleasant to take, as well as efficient. It must not, however, be used continuously.

Vitalia contains nourishment in the most concentrated form. It is valuable as a restorative and stimulant as well as a nutrient.

Bovinine is another preparation of beef of great value. It is in a form to be absorbed almost immediately without digestive effort.

Brand's beef jelly is the next best thing to good home-made beef-tea.

Liebig's beef-tea is more of a stimulant than a nutrient. But if taken with biscuit it is nourishing.

Among Milk preparations *Horlick's Malted Milk* is one of the most valuable. It is in dry powdered form, and can be mixed with either hot or cold water, requiring no cooking.

The various invalid foods are almost all good. Neave's, Ridge's and Du Barry's Revalenta (which consists chiefly of lentil flour, and may be replaced by the lentil flour itself) have obtained well-deserved reputations.

In dieting dyspestics the most important thing is the times of eating; next in importance is the quantity they take, most dyspeptics taking either too much or too little; and last, and less important than either of these two, is the regulation of the quality.

CHAPTER VII.

MATERIA MEDICA.

THERE is another way of classifying the different kinds of dyspepsia besides the one I have adopted above—that is, by taking the leading feature of each case. There are thus--*flatulent* dyspepsia, *painful* dyspepsia, *acid* dyspepsia, and many others. A division of this kind would cut through the classification I have already given, as examples of all these could be taken from any one of the kinds I have described. I have, therefore, decided to add this chapter of

Materia Medica, giving under each drug the particular symptoms which indicate its use in indigestion. By looking through the list of drugs I have given, the various dyspepsias—flatulent, acid, and the rest—will find their counterparts described. The medicines are arranged in alphabetical order, and only those characteristic symptoms which indicate the medicines in cases of dyspepsia are given.

Dose.—Unless otherwise stated, the dose of each medicine named should be one drop in water or on a small piece of sugar, or two pilules, of the 3d attenuation. It should be taken about an hour or half an hour before each meal.

Abies nigra.—Loss of appetite

in the morning, but great craving for food at noon and night. Severe pain in the stomach after eating; sensation as if an undigested hard boiled egg were there.

Actæa racemosa (also called *Cimicifuga racemosa*).—Great depression of spirits and feeling as if under a cloud. Severe headache, with aching in eyeballs. Unpleasant taste in mouth, unpleasant breath, nausea, sinking faintness at pit of stomach, vomiting. Tea dyspepsia.

Antimonium crudum. — Milky white tongue, or thickly coated tongue; eructations of wind, and fluid tasting of the food taken.

Antimonium tartaricum.—Milky white tongue; nausea; vomiting and prostration; tremulousness. Useful in the dyspepsia of drunkards.

Argentum nitricum.—Flatulent dyspepsia—the flatulence coming away easily and in great quantity. Great pain and tenderness at the stomach-pit, the pain being worse after any food. Palpitation and short breath; anæmia. This medicine is especially useful in anæmic girls, and also for flatulent dyspepsia resulting from eating cold food. Threatened ulceration of the stomach.

Arsenicum.—Irritable state of digestive mucous membrane. (Red tongue, or red with thin, white silvery coat); thirst; burning pain at the stomach; faintness; nausea, and vomiting. The bowels are generally loose; there is a low feverish state; wasting; anxiety; restlessness.

This medicine is useful in ulceration of the stomach, and in all cases of irritative dyspepsia with great vital exhaustion and depression.

Baptisia.—When there is great dulness and heaviness approaching the typhoid type, tongue foul, no appetite, often vomiting and diarrhœa. The head is heavy, and the face has a heavy expression. This medicine is very useful in indigestion after overloading the stomach, and in those acute attacks of indigestion with fever which used to be called "gastric fever" or "gastric attacks."

Bryonia.—Feeling as of a stone

at the pit of the stomach; sharp pain going through from this region to the back; pain between the shoulders or under one shoulder-blade; pain across the forehead; bilious vomiting; white tongue; constipation; stools large and light-coloured in rheumatic patients.

Bryonia is useful in many kinds of dyspepsia. An example has been given of its efficacy in the case of an arsenical dyspepsia. But its range is very wide, and any case presenting two or three of the above symptoms will be cured by the remedy.

Calcarea carbonica 6.—Acid dyspepsia; everything turning to acid; sour risings and eructations; heartburn; waterbrash; milk disagrees;

offensive white stools; useful in almost all cases where acidity is the leading feature. It is often of remarkable service in those cases where dyspepsia is premonitory of consumption of the lungs.

Carbo veg. 6.—Flatulent dyspepsia; great belching of wind; cutting pains in the chest; acidity; bowels regular or loose; gouty dyspepsia.

Carbo veg. is perhaps the most useful of all medicines in flatulent dyspepsia. The flatulence is chiefly in the stomach and passing away upwards. It is contrasted with *Lycopodium*, which has abdominal flatulence with constipation.

Carbolic acid.—Acute dyspepsia; great flatulence, passing upwards;

pains in the chest and stomach after all food ; nausea ; vomiting ; depression. There is usually a good deal of nervousness connected with the cases which call for *Carbolic acid.* It is good for nervous dyspepsia, *i.e.*, dyspepsia where nervous symptoms predominate.

Chamomilla.— Fretfulness and irritability are the leading indications for this remedy in whatever disease calls for it. It is especially called for in the dyspepsia of teething children. The special dyspeptic symptoms are:—Fulness of upper abdomen ; belching of wind ; pressure at the stomach as from a stone ; burning at the stomach ; irritable gastralgia ; windy colic ; green, watery or mucous diarrhœa ;

biliousness. Bitter taste in the mouth in the morning. Desire for acids, and thirst.

China.—Dyspepsia after exhausting diseases or vicious habits; dyspepsia of nervous debility; loss of appetite; loathing of food; shuddering and chilliness; heartburn; pressure at the stomach; nausea; vomiting; pain in the liver; light stools. When given in the $^{\theta}$ tincture it lessens the craving for alcohol.

Hydrastis Canadensis.—"Goneness" or sinking sensation after meals; yellow slimy tongue; sour or putrid eructations; alternate diarrhœa and constipation.

Ignatia.—Indigestion with nervous symptoms; sinking at the pit of the stomach; sensation of a lump in the throat. When indigestion is brought on or aggravated by worry. Aggravation by tobacco smoke. Stomach symptoms generally relieved by eating. Hysterical symptoms with indigestion.

Iodine.—Dyspepsia with great wasting. The appetite may be ravenous or absent. In dyspepsia from nervous causes, where there is complete failure of appetite, if *Iodine* is given in 3^x strength for half to a quarter of an hour before meal-times, it will often enable the patient to eat.

Ipecacuanha.—Sick dyspepsia; constant nausea; accumulation of saliva in the mouth; loss of appetite; sensation as if the stomach hung down relaxed.

Kali bichromicum.—Indigestion alternating with rheumatic symptoms; vomiting; gastritis; chronic catarrh of the stomach; tongue coated yellow, red beneath; weight rather than pain after food; dyspepsia of beer drinkers.

Lycopodium 6.—Flatulent distension of the bowels; flatulence passing downwards; rumbling; cannot bear the pressure of the clothes; waterbrash; tongue coated white; constipation; urine depositing a sediment; sleepiness after dinner in gouty patients.

Mercurius solubilis 6. — Pale flabby tongue; depraved taste; foul breath; light stools; depression of spirits.

Natrum muriaticum 6.—Bitter

taste in the mouth; waterbrash; heartburn; chilliness; palpitation after food; anæmia; constipation; useful in anæmic girls; also in youths who have indulged in evil habits.

Nux vomica.—From indigestible food; from beer, wine, or spirits; from tobacco; from excesses of all kinds. Suited to spare, swarthy persons of irascible temperament; tongue brown at the back; cramping or spasmodic pains; flatulence; vomiting; constipation.

Petroleum.—Constant sickness, and loathing of all food; bilious vomiting; breathlessness and bloodlessness; "green sickness."

Plumbum 6.—Cramping contracting pains in body and limbs, with indigestion. Obstinate constipation with colic. Sensation of a ball rising up from the stomach into the throat.

Pulsatilla. — From fat food; mucous derangement; thickly coated, moist, white tongue; nausea with little vomiting; heartburn; absence of much pain; feeling of distension; clothes have to be loosened; bowels loose or regular; suited to persons inclined to be stout, fair, and of a mild disposition.

Sulphur.—In chronic cases generally, where dyspepsia has followed the disappearance of a skin eruption; pressure and heaviness in the stomach after eating a little, and sour or empty eructations;

"sinking" sensation about 11 A. M.; bitter taste in the mouth; tongue coated white; griping about the navel; constipation; rheumatic and gouty dyspepsia. *Sulphur* is complementary to *Nux vomica*, they often do well in alternation.